Reversing Neutropenia: Testimonies of Hope. From Patients with Different Diseases Part 1

The Raw Vegan Plant-Based Detoxification & Regeneration Workbook for Healing Patients.

Volume 6

Health Central

Copyright © 2020

All rights reserved. Without limiting rights under the copyright reserved above, no part of this publication may be reproduced, stored, introduced into a retrieval system, distributed or transmitted in any form or by any means, including without limitation photocopying, recording, or other electronic or mechanical methods, without the prior written permission of the publisher, except in the case of brief quotations embodied in critical reviews and certain other non-commercial uses permitted by copyright law.

This book, with the opinions, suggestions and references made within it, is based on the author's personal experience and is for personal study and research purposes only. This program is about health and vitality, not disease. The author makes no medical claims. If you choose to use the material in this book on yourself, the author and publisher take no responsibility for your actions and decisions or the consequences thereof..

The scanning, uploading, and/or distribution of this document via the internet or via any other means without the permission of the publisher is illegal and is punishable by law. Please purchase only authorized editions and do not participate in or encourage electronic piracy of copyrightable materials

Important Information: a testimony tells a personal story, the information broadcast is published in a purely informative way and cannot be considered as medical recommendations. Testimonies are not a substitute for consultations, treatments or diagnosis from health professionals who have been certified with the health authorities. Testimonies do not promote any diet in particular, but simply illustrates the self-healing ability of the body when it meets its vital and physiological needs.

Topics Discussed & Journal Structure

1. Points Discussed In The Previous Volume

2. Testimonials & Success Stories

3. Important Notes for Overcoming Your Neutropenia

4. The Power of Journaling

5. Daily Journal Examples

6. 30 Day Assisted Journal Section

Points Discussed in Volume 5:

1 – Where does internal dysfunction stem from?

2 – What happens when the kidneys stop filtering effectively?

3 – Environmental factors that contribute to dis-ease.

4 – Why hydration is so important.

5 – Managing internal pH levels for better health.

6 – The adrenal gland and kidney connection.

7 – How best to achieve results? Fast – or – slow & steady?

Testimonials & Success Stories

Within this volume and the next volume we will be presenting you with a series of success stories from patients that have had a variety of chronic conditions and overcame them using the protocol that we have discussed in previous volumes. Our intention by sharing these testimonials is to give you hope and to realise that all of the information that we have discussed in our series thus far has worked across multiple different conditions, and therefore irrespective of the condition label, we have found this protocol to work for every case we have come across, including our very own conditions.

As mentioned in previous volumes, the root cause of all "disease" is the same, regardless of the name/label that has been given to it – and this is merely an accumulation of mucus and congestion within the blood/various organ(s), due to a continued intake of acid-forming foods. Your genetics, environment and lifestyle may also contribute to this, but for now, our focus is on your daily food intake.

With all diseases having the same root cause (acid, congestion, mucus) we rarely differentiate between the wide variety of labelled "diseases" in existence today. However, during treatment we do identify the main specific areas of weakness and address these directly with the use of herbs (and possibly various organ glandular meat/formulas), whilst the raw fruit and intermittent fasting routine is applied. The basic essence of curing the body is the same – i.e. flush out the stagnant acidic accumulated waste from the lymphatic system, through the kidneys (and colon), and as the body's health, alkalinity, and oxygen levels increase – witness it excel and self-heal through a raw vegan (predominantly fruit) dietary regimen.

Those who persist with this protocol and see it through to the end – regardless of the disease label they have been aligned with, will see a reversal of their condition eventually. However, each person is different and so there is no defined timescale for how long it will take to get better. We advise that you make this your new routine and put your aspirations of achieving results to one side. The ultimate goal is to increase your health to a higher level so that it can overpower and rid your body of any imbalances that it may be harbouring. You will experience a difference within yourself quite early on but this is not a sign that you have been healed – you must continue until there are no more signs of your condition.

Through reading these success stories, the key to look out for is the similarities in the protocols used – regardless of the challenge that was being faced. You will notice that the daily routine followed for curing and reversing any of these conditions is similar across the board, and you will pick up on this as you read the success stories. In the end, our goal is to stop consuming acid-forming foods (and cooked foods), and replace them with live electrical, high energy, alkaline raw fruit (coupled with intermittent dry fasting).

Note: We have removed any personal information and names from the following success stories for the purposes of privacy but the key details have been made available for your benefit and to take inspiration from. Everything is possible but you must focus and persist.

Success Story #1: Autoimmune Disease – Vitiligo (the supposedly "incurable autoimmune disease" and one of the "hardest to reverse")

"5 years ago I started to develop white patches on my skin, and this quickly spread across my back and face. I could not understand where it had come from because I felt that I lived quite a healthy lifestyle (constantly in the gym and eating the diet of a bodybuilder!). Any medical doctor that I went to see about it assured me that there was no cure for this condition which they called Vitiligo, a so-called autoimmune disease of the skin. The difficult challenge when seeing a medical doctor is that we give them so much authority that in the end, we start to buy into anything that they state or suggest. The reality however is that they are "symptom managers" and not "cure managers". I was offered plenty of UV light treatments along with some creams but these were merely symptom management tools, nothing for curing the root cause and ridding it out of my body forever.

Now that I knew that the medical community could not help, I started experimenting with a series of different diets, including the ketogenic diet, the carnivore diet, the cooked vegan diet, the Paleo diet and the Mediterranean Diet. Nothing worked. In fact my Vitiligo continued to spread.

I then came across this fruitarian lifestyle and was advised that we as human-beings were predominantly meant to be mainly fruit eaters with some vegetables, and the diet intended for us was to be raw, grown from the land, without any influences by man, just like it is for the other species in existence today.

This diet felt very natural and made sense to me so I started following the protocol of fasting (18+ hours) and eating nothing but fruit, my favourite being watermelons, mangos and litchi fruit. The immediate difference that I experienced was: increased urges and regularity behind my bowel movements and urination. The next thing I noticed was that my visits to the bathroom were always such ghastly smelling affairs. In short, I could feel the old trapped garbage being loosened up and offloaded with the help of my intermittent fasting and fruit diet. I did feel slightly hungry at times but then I would make myself a salad with my favourite vegetables (cucumber, tomato, lettuce, a few jalepeno chillis, bell peppers, with lemon juice and sesame seed paste being the salad dressing, or avocados if available).

Although I was having some success, my progress seemed slow until I found myself on a visit to Morocco! My results just accelerated here. I could not understand what was happening. My original skin colour was coming back very fast and the re-pigmentation felt miraculous. Then I had the following realisations:

1 - We were in a hot country which made me sweat out toxins.

2 - The sun was very dense in its presence and I could feel my body healing the more time I spent underneath it. I had previously been vitamin D deficient.

3 – I would visit the beach regularly and perform deep breathing exercises as I sat in front of the Mediterranean Sea (and the Atlantic Ocean). It felt like this fresh Oxygen was entering my cells and encouraging my body to heal.

4 – The fruit in Morocco was all organic, tree ripened and sweet. I had not really tasted such fruit in the UK. It was a joy to eat and felt like my body absorbed it so easily.

Within weeks, I started noticing my skin coloured spots re-appearing within the white patches on my body. They were populating in their masses and I was just left speechless at the power of this protocol. Whereas previously I had my doubts, I was now a believer in this high fruit diet. The results continued to be positive and now skip to present day (6 months on, back in the UK), of the remaining white patches, I am still seeing them slowly be re-pigmented and disappear. The fruit is not always the best here but you will get a good variety at any point in the year. I may return to Morocco or another country with hot weather and good fruit very soon, but until then I am happy making the most of what I currently have available to me. A huge thank you to God for allowing me to follow this path and discover this knowledge."

Success Story #2: Spinal Injury

"I suffered a spinal injury in 2007, compounded by a spinal birth defect. I spent years in a wheelchair or using a cane. I finally got sick of being told I'd never move normally again and taking 2 dozen pills a day. I went organic, cut meat consumption to a couple small portions a week, switched to herbal replacements for most of my meds, and started using reverse osmosis alkali water instead of tap water.

I haven't been in a wheelchair in 3 years. I put my cane away last July, and I walk 3-5 miles at least 3 times a week. And can even manage a short uphill sprint sometimes. I still have my nerve pain pills daily because I haven't found an adequate natural replacement. But I'm off everything else. I haven't lost weight because I'm regaining muscle from 11 years of immobility. But I've dropped 6-8 inches off my waist and down to a medium or large shirt from a 2x or 3x. A more natural approach is the only way to heal when all docs do these days are treat symptoms instead of the cause.

I share my journey with anyone who I think would benefit. If it helps just one person who has lost hope like I did, then it is worth it. And though my story is a good testimony, what it did for my husband is a better one.

The first year after I started making changes, he got very sick. He was in the intensive care unit in 2015 dying from glucose levels over 200, type 2 diabetes brought on by Statin use. I put him on a fruit diet similar to mine, and herbal remedies instead of meds and within a year had him off his insulin, blood pressure meds, and cholesterol meds. He's been medicine free for almost 3 years and his blood sugar and blood pressure have remained stable. He hasn't stuck with it, but I no longer fear for his health. There are so many cures for ailments in nature, but we've all been led to believe that doctors and pharmaceuticals are the only way to heal.

I spent 11 years in agony, with no doctor able to help. In the beginning, only sleeping an hour or two when my body gave out from exhaustion, waking a short while later from the pain. The first year I lived on maybe two dozen hours of sleep a week. Going back to the natural treatments I used earlier in life was the best decision I ever made. My journey isn't over yet, but I no longer believe it isn't possible."

Success Story #3: Cancer

"I'M OFFICIALLY CANCER FREE!

In 2017 I was diagnosed with cancer cells in my body (I won't go into the detail of where). I was getting treated in the Czech Republic, not America. I took several flights out there to follow up with my tests. I had one surgery last year that didn't work and it didn't get better, I said no to a second surgery because I didn't believe in knives cutting into my body anymore.

I remember I pre-recorded my dance classes and played it on a projector for the students overseas because I couldn't dance for 2 months after the surgery and my flights were already bought. I believed there's another way to heal myself. I immediately changed my whole living, eating and mental lifestyle around. I was in the depth of the study every day about holistic and natural herbal healing, Chinese medicine, alkaline raw veganism, different plants, herbs and water fasting.

In the end, I starved this cancer to death. Thank you [Name Removed] for being there for me and even doing the water fast with me & my friends and family always having my back. I'm celebrating my first day cancer free with a juice fast! I'm really thankful for this experience because without it I would continue putting trash into my body and trust me, it's not worth it. Earth heals."

Success Story #4: Lyme Disease - Candida

"This was a tough one to write. So many bad memories, but now filled with gratitude for how far I've come in 6 months.

Words cannot describe my gratitude to those who have been my healing guides along the way. You have helped save my life and I will be eternally grateful. Also, thanks to my husband who has walked through the fire with me on my darkest days.

And here's my story...

January 15, 2019 was the 6 month marker for starting on the raw fruit diet. I have been sick for many years, searching daily for the answers to get well. The last three years, I was pretty much bound to the house and not able to function well enough to be part of the world.

First I ended up in the hospital with an allergic reaction, struggling for life. After this point, I followed this raw fruit protocol for 6 months and on our 40th anniversary trip to Mexico, I was celebrating my newfound life.

I saw countless physicians who gave me up for crazy or hopeless, natural healers, naturopaths, tried almost every therapy possible, stayed in healing clinics out of state for up to 3 weeks, tried practically every diet possible, took thousands of supplements, flown across the country and even overseas to find answers. I had to be flown to Florida from my home state of Illinois 4 - 5 times to have good bacteria put in my intestines so I didn't die.

And nothing worked...

... and then that moment that everything changes.

One night I got my mind quiet with meditating and afterwards felt strongly I needed to post on a particular online group. I never would have guessed this post would lead me to the truth and healing I was seeking. Someone who cared enough to take the time to give me some information about this raw fruit protocol. At first I dismissed it. Who wants to be told that their thinking about their current protocol is wrong, we've all been there, right?

Thank goodness the next day I was led back to the post and chose to pursue this path further. Immediately I felt that this information resonated with my soul and that THIS is the answer I had been praying for. It totally made sense.

That very day I told my husband, "let's go buy some fruit" and I've never looked back or questioned the protocol.

With an ambiguous diagnosis of Lyme Disease, anxiety, flesh eating bacteria, life-threatening intestinal bacteria, mold toxicity, Candida and so much more, I struggled every day to live for so many years. My everyday existence was all about surviving, that's all. I had to spend countless hours each day treating the symptoms so my body wasn't overcome by it all.

Keep in mind, this is just a short synopsis of my story. There's so much more to tell and my plan is to write a book in order to give others hope that they too can overcome.

The great news is now... today, I am finally healing and getting better daily. The fruit diet has enabled my body to detox the Lymph system and to get my kidneys filtering out all the disgusting bacteria, toxins, parasites, etc. By clearing out the gunk, the truth has been exposed which has me continuing on this crazy, amazing healing journey.

So here I am writing this from a hotel room in Phoenix, Arizona where I am on a business trip with my husband, engaging in activities, meetings, dinners and social events with about 1000 other people who are in an elite class of financial advisors. It's hard to imagine that I could not even leave the house 6 months ago. Gratitude fills my entire being for those who took the time to guide me this information on such a dark, scary night 6 months ago.

Am I completely well? No, not at all. It takes time to detox a 59 year old body that has been collecting and storing toxins for all these years.

Am I considerably better? You betcha! I have a life now and no longer wake up every day wondering if I will survive the day. Instead I look forward to a future of incredible health and vitality and a knowingness my best days are ahead because I've never been healthy my entire life. And if I'm healthy, I can do it all, enjoying a life full of adventure, freedom and abundance.

Do I believe I could become well instantaneously? Absolutely! The mind is powerful and the body will act according to our thoughts, emotions and beliefs. I won't give up until I can gain control over this.

Although I do not focus on symptoms at all these days, but instead keeping my mindset on my amazing future and gratitude for the present moment, I have posted my previous symptoms below that have been healed or almost healed to give others encouragement and hope. Keep in mind this is a short list of everything I had going on:

Muscle tightness in neck, head and shoulders so much so my head was drawn to the side and I could not hold it straight or turn one way or another.

Debilitating Fatigue - could hardly walk from one side of the house to the other.

Flesh eating MRSA for 5+ years on several places on different parts of my body - a constant fear my ears and other body parts would be completely eaten away.

C-diff intestinal infection that required many trips to the ER and to Florida to replenish the good bacteria. This infection kills 50% of the people who have it each year.

Horrible brain fog, inability to make decisions, think clearly. Sometimes I hardly knew who I was or where I was.

Hypothyroidism - I am no longer taking thyroid medication or any medication.

Anxiety was through the roof with an overwhelming sense that I was going to die at any time.

I think I had the worse parasite infection on the face of the earth (still treating, but much better).

Pounding heart 24/7. I could hear my heartbeat in right ear constantly.

Eyes blurring, painful, twitching, extreme dryness. Pulsating and flashing in eyes.

Pain and heaviness in lungs. Rib cage pain. Daily intestinal pain.

Movement throughout skin (now I know this is scabies - and it's better but still present)

Stagnant lymph system - tests constantly coming back with reports of heavy metals, high chemical, pesticide load, mold toxicity, mycotoxins, etc.

Kidneys not filtering - edema in legs (doctor in the ER told me this was normal).

Sad and depressed and cried every day (now I can't imagine feeling like that). Terrified to be alone.

Thoughts consumed with concern over whether I would get better.

Constant rashes and hives. Low blood pressure. Always cold, often had chills.

So there are more symptoms, but you get the picture. I am lucky to be alive.... I take that back. The only reason I am alive is because I believed in my heart of hearts that God had a purpose for me and if I kept researching, experimenting and believing I would someday figure it out. And I did!

I am so thankful to have discovered this way of life and all my fruitarian friends that I have bumped into and who have helped guide me along the way!

I can't attribute my healing totally to the diet though. It's so much more. Now I know we are creators of our own lives and I am always in control of my health through my thoughts and emotions.

My purpose here is to give you hope. For those of you who are in the heat of the battle, know there is an answer and the choice is yours to heal yourself as I am doing. It's always a choice. And then the difficult part begins, putting it into action even when the future seems bleak and there is yet no evidence that is working. Surround yourself with those who have walked the path before you and found success. There are many communities and teachers out there that will guide you in the diet and help you find the power of the mind and to rid yourself of destructive programs that are holding you back.

Keep educating yourself.

It's so important to let go of the victimhood and open yourself to possibility of healing because you are worth it and you deserve it. NEVER GIVE UP!

Healing is always possible! If we take out what doesn't serve us and put in what does, the body will heal itself miraculously. Be free and love yourself. Feel free to share with those who might need hope!"

The second part to these Success Stories continues in the next volume.

If you have a success story to share, please feel free to email it to us at: **healingcentral8@gmail.com**

Wishing you all the best.

Our Story

It was a Sunday night, over 7 years ago – I was in bed – tossing and turning – unable to sleep. I watched the time pass, from 11pm, to 12am... to 1:30am. I just couldn't sleep. I could feel an immense pressure in my chest cavity and all across my diaphragm area. I couldn't understand where this was coming from. I got up and had some water, I then tried to use the bathroom – the discomfort was still there. Nothing seemed to work – I felt like I was being suffocated each time I would lie down. In the end, I fell asleep out of sheer fatigue.

At the time, I was a sufferer of asthma, eczema, anxiety attacks, and a damaged/leaky gut. These conditions had lead to many symptoms that doctors could not offer me any answers for. I had many tests done but nothing could tell me what the root causes of my problems were.

I started researching about my symptoms, and as I did this, I found myself expanding into the area of medical history. As my research continued, I came to understand that our ancestors lived healthy and long lives, without the health challenges of today.

Eventually, I stumbled upon a few health forums which I joined. Through these, I met a series of individuals that were battling a variety of conditions themselves (a rare genetic disorder, Crohn's disease, multiple sclerosis, muscular dystrophy (MD), diabetes, cushing's disease, a series of 'incurable' autoimmune diseases, and cancer).

We all came together and as we started to grow as a group, we made a significant discovery - that actually the cure to all diseases was discovered back in the 1920s by a Dr Arnold Ehret.

As we studied his material, we started applying his information and protocols on ourselves. This seemed like one experiment worth trying, and within 2 weeks, regardless of our individual conditions, we all started to notice a difference in our improved digestion, higher energy levels, increased mental clarity and improved physical ability. A major change was taking place – our health was improving, as our conditions were decreasing.

We continued to expand our knowledge and we started to encounter even more communities and learnt that there were more magnificent and very gifted healers out there. We came across the works and achievements of Dr Sebi, and completed an insightful and very informative course by Dr Robert Morse.

The essential message of these great healers was very similar to that of Dr Arnold Ehret. Now we had even further confirmation that the information we had been following thus far was in fact THE path to health success. With our progress so far, we could sense victory.

Within 3 months, 30 to 40 percent of our symptoms had disappeared and our health was becoming stronger. Some of us started to take specific herbs in order to enhance the detoxification.

Another 3 months on and the majority of us no longer experienced any more symptoms. Our blood work had also improved significantly, but we still had work to do in order to completely heal.

Now that we had made significant progress in reversing our conditions through self-experimentation, we started to offer basic healthy eating advice to the sick within our local communities.

Eventually, we started working with local patients on a voluntary basis. It was heartbreaking to witness lives being cut short or chronic sickness being accepted as a way of life – all whilst the lifelong eating habits of these individuals remained. The most common diseases that we were coming across included: cancers, heart disease, chronic kidney disease, high blood pressure, varying infections, and diabetes.

By helping our communities with changing their daily eating habits, we started seeing results, and although the transitional phase of moving from the foods that they were so used to eating, to moving over to a raw plant-based routine was a challenge, in the end, it was worth the shift. Note: there were many that ignored our advice and sadly they continued to remain in their state.

We did have resistance initially from family members and friends of the sick but after some time as they started seeing health improvements, more started joining us, and they also started experiencing what we had when we first set out on our journey of natural self-healing.

Nevertheless, challenges still remained – the main ones being the undoing of society's programming that cooked food is an essential part of life (including animal and wheat based products) and raw food alone surely cannot be good for you. It doesn't take long to explain how to remove imbalances and dis-ease from within the human body but the more extensive task is to actually have the protocol information applied and adhered to completely.

This is where the idea for this series of journal & progress tracker stemmed from. We felt compelled to spread this information in a more digestible and applicable form, over a series of volumes, in which we would start by offering some key informative points, followed by a journal which would allow for you to actually apply the information, record your progress, daily feelings and stay accountable to yourself. We also found that journaling and writing to oneself really helps to self-motivate and enhances a self consciousness that is needed when following a protocol like this.

Each journal volume within this series will be designed to help you record your journey for a 30 day period. At the start of each journal we will continue to offer insightful information about our experiences, whilst expanding on and re-iterating specific parts of this protocol.

The fact that you are reading this foreword is an indication that you are already on your way to self-healing. Regardless of your condition, we invite you to seek more knowledge and set your health free.

May you always remain blessed and guided.

Much Love From The Health Central Team

Important Notes for Overcoming Your Neutropenia

1. It should be noted that based on our experiences and understanding, whether your condition is Neutropenia, or any other, we recommend the same raw vegan healing protocol across all spectrums. With some conditions, you may need to perform a deeper detoxification (using herbs - or organ/glandular meat/capsules for more chronic situations) before achieving significant results, but in general, we have found this protocol to work in most cases. In our experience, the goal is not to cure, but instead to raise health levels first, through healthy food choices, as intended for our species – before the eradication and prevention of these modern-day "disease" conditions can take place.

2. With all conditions, we have found that the lymphatic system has become congested and overwhelmed due to the kidneys not efficiently filtering out the accumulated cell waste – as a result of years of dehydrating cooked/wheat/dairy foods. The adrenal glands work closely with the kidneys, and so adrenal/kidney herbs and glandular formulas played a major role in opening up these channels. We also found that opening up the bowels and loosening the gut was hugely important too.

3. The healing protocol that we used on ourselves is discussed and expanded upon throughout the various volumes in this series. Our goal is to share information that we have gathered from our journeys, and let you decide if it is something that you feel could also work for you in your

journey for health and vitality. You are not obliged to use this information, and you may proceed as you see fit.

Through our study, research and application, we have found this system to correct any internal imbalances and remove dis-ease that has occurred within the human body, due to the continued consumption of acid-forming foods.

4. Always take progression ultra slow and go at your own pace. Listen to your body at every stage. We cannot re-iterate this point enough. Pay attention to how you feel and continue to consult your doctor and monitor your blood work.

5. A special emphasis needs to be given to the transition phase when moving from your regular, standard diet, to a raw vegan diet that is high in fruit. You must take your time and slowly remove foods from your current routine, and replace them with either fasting or a small amount of fruit in the initial stages. Work with small amounts – please do not make any drastic changes. If you do not feel comfortable or have any concerns at any stage, please immediately stop.

Note: with any dietary change, this can be a stressful event for the body and so it is important that you support your kidneys and adrenal glands using the appropriate herbs and glandular formulas previously mentioned.

6. Before partaking in any new dietary routine, please always consult your Doctor first and ensure that they are aware of your health related goals. This approach is beneficial because (a) you can monitor your blood work with your doctor as you progress with this new protocol, and (b) if you are on any medication, as your health improves, you

can review its need and/or discuss having dosage amounts reduced (if necessary).

7. Please note that we are sharing information from our collective experiences of how we healed ourselves from a variety of diseases and conditions. These are solely our own opinions. Having reversed a range of conditions using essentially the same protocol, our understanding and conclusion, based on our experience alone, is that regardless of the disease, illness or condition name – removing it from the human body stems from correcting your diet and transitioning over to a more raw vegan lifestyle.

8. Proceed with care, and again, do not make any sudden changes – always take your time in slowly removing foods that are not serving you, and replacing them with high energy sweet tree-ripened juicy fruit. If at any point you feel that you are moving too quickly, please adjust your transition accordingly. Results may vary between individuals.

9. We recommended that you constantly expand your knowledge and familiarise yourself with the works of Dr Arnold Ehret, Dr Robert Morse and John Rose. When you feel confident with your understanding, start taking gradual steps towards reaching your goals. Make the most of this journal and use it to serve you as a companion on your journey.

The Power of Journaling

a) Journaling your inner self talk is a truly effective way of increasing self awareness and consciousness. To be able to transfer your thoughts and feelings onto a piece of paper is a truly effective method of self reflection and improvement. This is much needed when you are switching to a high fruit dietary routine.

b) Be sure to always add the date of journaling at the top of each page used. This is invaluable for when you wish to go back and review/track progress and your feelings/thoughts on previous dates.

c) Keep a comprehensive record of activities, thoughts, and really log everything you ate/are eating. You can even make miscellaneous notes if you feel that they will help you.

d) We have added tips and questions to offer you guidance, reminders, inspiration and areas to journal about.

e) We like to use journals to have a conversation with ourselves. Inner talk can really help you overcome any challenges that you are experiencing. Express yourself and any concerns that you may have.

f) Try to advise yourself as though you are your best friend – similarly to how you would advise a close friend or family member. You will be surprised at the results that you will achieve from using this technique.

g) Add notes to this journal and work your way through the 30 days. Once completed, move onto the next journal volume in this series, which will also be structured in a similar, supportive and educational fashion. We have produced a series of these journals in order to cater for your ongoing journey and goals.

h) For those of you who would like to track your progress with a more basic notebook-style journal, we have produced a separate series in which each notebook interior differs. This is to cater for your complete health journaling needs.

We have laid out the following examples to serve as potential frameworks for one way of how a journal could be filled in on a daily basis. These are just basic examples, but you can complete your daily journals in any other way that you feel is most comfortable and effective for you.

[EXAMPLE 1]
Today's Date: 3rd Jan 2020

Morning
Dry fasting (water and food free since 8pm last night) - will go up until 12:30pm today, and start with 500ml of spring water before eating half a watermelon.

Afternoon
Kept busy and was in and out quite a bit - so nothing consumed.

Evening
At around 5pm, I had a peppermint tea with a selection of mixed dried fruit (small bowl of apricot, dates, mango, pineapple, and prunes).

Night
Sipped on spring water through the evening as required.
Finished off the other half of the watermelon from the morning.

Today's Notes (Highlights, Thoughts, Feelings):

As with most days, today started well with me dry fasting (continuing my fast from my sleep/skipping breakfast) up until around 12:30pm and then eating half a watermelon. The laxative effect of the watermelon helped me poop and release any loosened toxins from the fasting period.
I tend to struggle on some days from 3pm onwards. Up until that point I am okay but if the cravings strike then it can be challenging. I remind myself that those burgers and chips do not have any live healing energy.
I feel good in general. I feel fantastic doing a fruit/juice fast but slightly empty by the end of the day.
Cooked food makes me feel severe fatigue and mental fog.
Will continue with my fruit fasting and start to introduce fruit juices due to their deeper detox benefits. I would love to be on juices only as I have seen others within the community achieve amazing results.

[EXAMPLE 2]
Today's Date: 4th Jan 2020

Morning

Today I woke and my children were enjoying some watermelon for breakfast - and the smell was luring so I joined them. Large bowl of watermelon eaten at around 8am. Started with a glass of water.

Afternoon

Snacked on left over watermelon throughout the morning and afternoon. Had 5 dates an hour or so after.

Evening

Had around 3 mangoes at around 6pm. Felt content - but then I was invited round to a family gathering where a selection of pizzas, burgers and chips were being served. I gave into the peer pressure and felt like I let myself down!

Night

Having over-eaten earlier on in the evening, I was still feeling bloated with a headache (possibly digestion related) and I also felt quite mucus filled (wheez in chest and coughing up phlegm). Very sleepy and low energy. The perils of cooked foods!!

Today's Notes (Highlights, Thoughts, Feelings):

I let myself down today. It all started well until I ate a fully blown meal (and over-ate). I didn't remain focussed and I spun off track. As a result my energy levels were much lower and I felt a bout of extreme fatigue 30 minutes after the meal (most likely the body struggling to with digesting all that cooked food).
I need to stick to the plan because the difference between fruit fasting, and eating cooked foods is huge - 1 makes you feel empowered whilst the other makes you feel drained. I also felt the mucus overload after the meal - it kicked in pretty quickly.
Today I felt disappointed after giving in to the meal but tomorrow is a new day and I will keep on going! It is important to remind myself that I won't get better if I cannot stick to the routine.

1. Today's Date:

Morning
(work towards continuing your night time dry fast up until at least 12pm)

Afternoon
(get hydrating with fresh fruit or even better slow juiced fruits/berries/melons)

Evening
(aim to wind down to a dry fast by around 6pm to 7pm)

Night
(work your way up to dry fasting from the evening until 12pm the following day)

Today's Notes (Highlights, Thoughts, Feelings, What Could You Improve On?)

"Get yourself an accountability partner to complete a 30 day detox with. Start with 7 days and work your way up. It will be fun and motivating completing it with somebody (or a group) ...or of course you can go it alone."

2. Today's Date:

—————————————— Morning ——————————————
(work towards continuing your night time dry fast up until at least 12pm)

—————————————— Afternoon ——————————————
(get hydrating with fresh fruit or even better slow juiced fruits/berries/melons)

—————————————— Evening ——————————————
(aim to wind down to a dry fast by around 6pm to 7pm)

—————————————— Night ——————————————
(work your way up to dry fasting from the evening until 12pm the following day)

Today's Notes (Highlights, Thoughts, Feelings, What Could You Improve On?)

"Remember when starting out, it is important to keep yourself hydrated throughout the day. Spring Water is a good start - and slow/cold pressed juice is also very powerful."

3. Today's Date:

————————————— Morning —————————————
(work towards continuing your night time dry fast up until at least 12pm)

————————————— Afternoon —————————————
(get hydrating with fresh fruit or even better slow juiced fruits/berries/melons)

————————————— Evening —————————————
(aim to wind down to a dry fast by around 6pm to 7pm)

————————————— Night —————————————
(work your way up to dry fasting from the evening until 12pm the following day)

Today's Notes (Highlights, Thoughts, Feelings, What Could You Improve On?)

"Eat melons/watermelons separately, and before any other fruit as it digests faster and we want to limit fermentation (acidity) which can occur if other fruits are mixed in."

4. Today's Date:

Morning
(work towards continuing your night time dry fast up until at least 12pm)

Afternoon
(get hydrating with fresh fruit or even better slow juiced fruits/berries/melons)

Evening
(aim to wind down to a dry fast by around 6pm to 7pm)

Night
(work your way up to dry fasting from the evening until 12pm the following day)

Today's Notes (Highlights, Thoughts, Feelings, What Could You Improve On?)

"Stay focussed on the end goal of removing mucus & toxins from your body and feeling wonderful! Look forward to being full of vitality and disease free once again"

5. Today's Date:

Morning
(work towards continuing your night time dry fast up until at least 12pm)

Afternoon
(get hydrating with fresh fruit or even better slow juiced fruits/berries/melons)

Evening
(aim to wind down to a dry fast by around 6pm to 7pm)

Night
(work your way up to dry fasting from the evening until 12pm the following day)

Today's Notes (Highlights, Thoughts, Feelings, What Could You Improve On?)

"Meditate and perform deep breathing exercises in order to help yourself remain present minded and on track. Perform these techniques throughout the day but also during any challenging times that you may come to face."

6. Today's Date:

Morning
(work towards continuing your night time dry fast up until at least 12pm)

Afternoon
(get hydrating with fresh fruit or even better slow juiced fruits/berries/melons)

Evening
(aim to wind down to a dry fast by around 6pm to 7pm)

Night
(work your way up to dry fasting from the evening until 12pm the following day)

Today's Notes (Highlights, Thoughts, Feelings, What Could You Improve On?)

"Join a few like-minded communities – there are many juicing and raw vegan based groups, both online and offline. Being part of a community can help motivate you to reach your goals. You will also learn a great amount from others. Seeing others succeed is empowering."

7. Today's Date:

Morning
(work towards continuing your night time dry fast up until at least 12pm)

Afternoon
(get hydrating with fresh fruit or even better slow juiced fruits/berries/melons)

Evening
(aim to wind down to a dry fast by around 6pm to 7pm)

Night
(work your way up to dry fasting from the evening until 12pm the following day)

Today's Notes (Highlights, Thoughts, Feelings, What Could You Improve On?)

"If you are struggling to cope with hunger pangs in the early stages, try some dates or dried apricots, prunes, or raisins, with a cup of herbal tea. However, these pangs will disappear once your body adjusts to your new routine."

8. Today's Date:

——————————— Morning ———————————
(work towards continuing your night time dry fast up until at least 12pm)

——————————— Afternoon ———————————
(get hydrating with fresh fruit or even better slow juiced fruits/berries/melons)

——————————— Evening ———————————
(aim to wind down to a dry fast by around 6pm to 7pm)

——————————— Night ———————————
(work your way up to dry fasting from the evening until 12pm the following day)

Today's Notes (Highlights, Thoughts, Feelings, What Could You Improve On?)

"Get into a routine of regularly buying fresh fruit (or grow your own if weather permits) to keep your supplies up. Local wholesale markets do also clear fruits/veg on Fridays (if they are closed for the weekend) at a lower price, so they are worth a visit."

9. Today's Date:

Morning
(work towards continuing your night time dry fast up until at least 12pm)

Afternoon
(get hydrating with fresh fruit or even better slow juiced fruits/berries/melons)

Evening
(aim to wind down to a dry fast by around 6pm to 7pm)

Night
(work your way up to dry fasting from the evening until 12pm the following day)

Today's Notes (Highlights, Thoughts, Feelings, What Could You Improve On?)

"Regularly remind yourself about the great rewards and benefits that you will experience by keeping up this detoxification process. Imagine the lives you could save as a result of healing yourself."

10. Today's Date:

Morning
(work towards continuing your night time dry fast up until at least 12pm)

Afternoon
(get hydrating with fresh fruit or even better slow juiced fruits/berries/melons)

Evening
(aim to wind down to a dry fast by around 6pm to 7pm)

Night
(work your way up to dry fasting from the evening until 12pm the following day)

Today's Notes (Highlights, Thoughts, Feelings, What Could You Improve On?)

"Keep your teeth brushed (using miswak; a natural brush). Use coconut oil to oil pull before bedtime. Done correctly, you will notice an improvement in your dental health with these practices."

11. Today's Date:

────────────────── **Morning** ──────────────────

(work towards continuing your night time dry fast up until at least 12pm)

────────────────── **Afternoon** ──────────────────

(get hydrating with fresh fruit or even better slow juiced fruits/berries/melons)

────────────────── **Evening** ──────────────────

(aim to wind down to a dry fast by around 6pm to 7pm)

────────────────── **Night** ──────────────────

(work your way up to dry fasting from the evening until 12pm the following day)

Today's Notes (Highlights, Thoughts, Feelings, What Could You Improve On?)

"Be motivated by the vision of becoming an example for others to learn from and follow. You could change the lives of family and friends by showing them your own improvements."

12. Today's Date:

——————————— Morning ———————————
(work towards continuing your night time dry fast up until at least 12pm)

——————————— Afternoon ———————————
(get hydrating with fresh fruit or even better slow juiced fruits/berries/melons)

——————————— Evening ———————————
(aim to wind down to a dry fast by around 6pm to 7pm)

——————————— Night ———————————
(work your way up to dry fasting from the evening until 12pm the following day)

Today's Notes (Highlights, Thoughts, Feelings, What Could You Improve On?)

"Embrace your achievements and wonderful results – feel and appreciate the difference within you as a result of this new routine. Notice how your personal agility and fitness has improved. Feel the improved energy levels."

13. Today's Date:

Morning
(work towards continuing your night time dry fast up until at least 12pm)

Afternoon
(get hydrating with fresh fruit or even better slow juiced fruits/berries/melons)

Evening
(aim to wind down to a dry fast by around 6pm to 7pm)

Night
(work your way up to dry fasting from the evening until 12pm the following day)

Today's Notes (Highlights, Thoughts, Feelings, What Could You Improve On?)

"Buy fruit in bulk where possible so you have ample supplies for a week or two in advance. If in a hot climate, you could even freeze your fruit or make ice lollies out of it (crush & freeze). Immerse yourself in fruit so it becomes your only option."

14. Today's Date:

———————————— Morning ————————————
(work towards continuing your night time dry fast up until at least 12pm)

———————————— Afternoon ————————————
(get hydrating with fresh fruit or even better slow juiced fruits/berries/melons)

———————————— Evening ————————————
(aim to wind down to a dry fast by around 6pm to 7pm)

———————————— Night ————————————
(work your way up to dry fasting from the evening until 12pm the following day)

Today's Notes (Highlights, Thoughts, Feelings, What Could You Improve On?)

"Stay as busy as you can during the daytime. Creating a busy routine makes it easier to manage your diet. Have a purpose, and keep setting yourself new tasks/actions in order to keep yourself occupied."

15. Today's Date:

Morning
(work towards continuing your night time dry fast up until at least 12pm)

Afternoon
(get hydrating with fresh fruit or even better slow juiced fruits/berries/melons)

Evening
(aim to wind down to a dry fast by around 6pm to 7pm)

Night
(work your way up to dry fasting from the evening until 12pm the following day)

Today's Notes (Highlights, Thoughts, Feelings, What Could You Improve On?)

"Complete your fruit and fasting routine with a group of friends/family/colleagues so you can all support one another. Make it fun - set challenges - dry fast together and break your fasts together - have weekly catch up sessions."

16. Today's Date:

Morning
(work towards continuing your night time dry fast up until at least 12pm)

Afternoon
(get hydrating with fresh fruit or even better slow juiced fruits/berries/melons)

Evening
(aim to wind down to a dry fast by around 6pm to 7pm)

Night
(work your way up to dry fasting from the evening until 12pm the following day)

Today's Notes (Highlights, Thoughts, Feelings, What Could You Improve On?)

"Look out for white cloud/sediment (acids) in your urine to confirm that your kidneys are filtering out waste. Urinate in a glass jar - leave for 2 hours to settle before observing."

17. Today's Date:

———————————— Morning ————————————
(work towards continuing your night time dry fast up until at least 12pm)

———————————— Afternoon ————————————
(get hydrating with fresh fruit or even better slow juiced fruits/berries/melons)

———————————— Evening ————————————
(aim to wind down to a dry fast by around 6pm to 7pm)

———————————— Night ————————————
(work your way up to dry fasting from the evening until 12pm the following day)

Today's Notes (Highlights, Thoughts, Feelings, What Could You Improve On?)

"Have genuine love and care for yourself. If you are craving junk food, affirm positive inner talk ("I won't feel good after eating junk. I love myself too much to put my body through that - so leave it out!"). You can also take Sea Kelp, Coconut Water, or Celery to reduce any salt cravings."

18. Today's Date:

Morning
(work towards continuing your night time dry fast up until at least 12pm)

Afternoon
(get hydrating with fresh fruit or even better slow juiced fruits/berries/melons)

Evening
(aim to wind down to a dry fast by around 6pm to 7pm)

Night
(work your way up to dry fasting from the evening until 12pm the following day)

Today's Notes (Highlights, Thoughts, Feelings, What Could You Improve On?)

"Feel and note down the difference within yourself as you filter out unwanted acids with this alkaline, water-dense high fruit protocol."

19. Today's Date:

Morning
(work towards continuing your night time dry fast up until at least 12pm)

Afternoon
(get hydrating with fresh fruit or even better slow juiced fruits/berries/melons)

Evening
(aim to wind down to a dry fast by around 6pm to 7pm)

Night
(work your way up to dry fasting from the evening until 12pm the following day)

Today's Notes (Highlights, Thoughts, Feelings, What Could You Improve On?)

"Look for acidic waste/sediments in your urine regularly in order to ensure your kidneys are filtering. Dry fasting for over 18 hours will increase kidney filtration. You can also drink the juice of slow-juiced citrus fruits (lemons, oranges). Sweating helps too."

20. Today's Date:

Morning
(work towards continuing your night time dry fast up until at least 12pm)

Afternoon
(get hydrating with fresh fruit or even better slow juiced fruits/berries/melons)

Evening
(aim to wind down to a dry fast by around 6pm to 7pm)

Night
(work your way up to dry fasting from the evening until 12pm the following day)

Today's Notes (Highlights, Thoughts, Feelings, What Could You Improve On?)

"Infections emerge in an acidic environment. In order to remove infections, you must concentrate on kidney filtration. Use herbs for kidneys and adrenal glands - using dry fasting to assist."

21. Today's Date:

Morning
(work towards continuing your night time dry fast up until at least 12pm)

Afternoon
(get hydrating with fresh fruit or even better slow juiced fruits/berries/melons)

Evening
(aim to wind down to a dry fast by around 6pm to 7pm)

Night
(work your way up to dry fasting from the evening until 12pm the following day)

Today's Notes (Highlights, Thoughts, Feelings, What Could You Improve On?)

"Any deficiencies that you may have will start to disappear once you have cleansed your congested gut/colon, kidneys and various other eliminative organs."

22. Today's Date:

Morning
(work towards continuing your night time dry fast up until at least 12pm)

Afternoon
(get hydrating with fresh fruit or even better slow juiced fruits/berries/melons)

Evening
(aim to wind down to a dry fast by around 6pm to 7pm)

Night
(work your way up to dry fasting from the evening until 12pm the following day)

Today's Notes (Highlights, Thoughts, Feelings, What Could You Improve On?)

"Dependant on how deeply you detoxify yourself, it is possible to eliminate any genetic weaknesses that you may have inherited. This will require a deep detoxification process which involves juicing your fruits with prolonged periods of dry fasting"

23. Today's Date:

Morning
(work towards continuing your night time dry fast up until at least 12pm)

Afternoon
(get hydrating with fresh fruit or even better slow juiced fruits/berries/melons)

Evening
(aim to wind down to a dry fast by around 6pm to 7pm)

Night
(work your way up to dry fasting from the evening until 12pm the following day)

Today's Notes (Highlights, Thoughts, Feelings, What Could You Improve On?)

"Stay focused on your detoxification for deeper, lasting results. All past injuries / trauma are also repairable for good. Get those old acids out and replace them with a pain-free alkaline environment"

24. Today's Date:

Morning
(work towards continuing your night time dry fast up until at least 12pm)

Afternoon
(get hydrating with fresh fruit or even better slow juiced fruits/berries/melons)

Evening
(aim to wind down to a dry fast by around 6pm to 7pm)

Night
(work your way up to dry fasting from the evening until 12pm the following day)

Today's Notes (Highlights, Thoughts, Feelings, What Could You Improve On?)

*"If you suffer from ongoing sadness / depression, a deep detox will support your mental health. You will soon notice a positive change in your mood. **Note:** you will need to support your adrenal glands and kidneys with glandulars and/or herbs (liqorice root, sea kelp, uva ursi, nettle)"*

25. Today's Date:

Morning
(work towards continuing your night time dry fast up until at least 12pm)

Afternoon
(get hydrating with fresh fruit or even better slow juiced fruits/berries/melons)

Evening
(aim to wind down to a dry fast by around 6pm to 7pm)

Night
(work your way up to dry fasting from the evening until 12pm the following day)

Today's Notes (Highlights, Thoughts, Feelings, What Could You Improve On?)

"Have your fruits/ juices throughout the day - with dry fasting gaps of at least 3 hours in-between each feed. As the evening approaches, start to dry fast fully – from this point on, your body wants to rest and heal."

26. Today's Date:

Morning
(work towards continuing your night time dry fast up until at least 12pm)

Afternoon
(get hydrating with fresh fruit or even better slow juiced fruits/berries/melons)

Evening
(aim to wind down to a dry fast by around 6pm to 7pm)

Night
(work your way up to dry fasting from the evening until 12pm the following day)

Today's Notes (Highlights, Thoughts, Feelings, What Could You Improve On?)

"The kidneys dislike proteins but really appreciate juicy fruits like melons, berries, citrus fruits, pineapples, mangoes, apples, grapes. Witness the difference by replacing cooked foods and protein with fruits. Become the change."

27. Today's Date:

Morning
(work towards continuing your night time dry fast up until at least 12pm)

Afternoon
(get hydrating with fresh fruit or even better slow juiced fruits/berries/melons)

Evening
(aim to wind down to a dry fast by around 6pm to 7pm)

Night
(work your way up to dry fasting from the evening until 12pm the following day)

Today's Notes (Highlights, Thoughts, Feelings, What Could You Improve On?)

"Healing is very easy. There's no need to complicate it. Keep everything simple and you will see results. Concentrate on improving your level of health to a point where dis-ease is dissolved"

28. Today's Date:

Morning
(work towards continuing your night time dry fast up until at least 12pm)

Afternoon
(get hydrating with fresh fruit or even better slow juiced fruits/berries/melons)

Evening
(aim to wind down to a dry fast by around 6pm to 7pm)

Night
(work your way up to dry fasting from the evening until 12pm the following day)

Today's Notes (Highlights, Thoughts, Feelings, What Could You Improve On?)

"Keep your body in an alkaline and hydrated state as this is where regeneration takes place - and disease cannot continue to exist. You can achieve this through a raw fruits and vegetables diet (find your balance between the two)"

29. Today's Date:

Morning
(work towards continuing your night time dry fast up until at least 12pm)

Afternoon
(get hydrating with fresh fruit or even better slow juiced fruits/berries/melons)

Evening
(aim to wind down to a dry fast by around 6pm to 7pm)

Night
(work your way up to dry fasting from the evening until 12pm the following day)

Today's Notes (Highlights, Thoughts, Feelings, What Could You Improve On?)

"An enema with boiled water (cooled down) can support your detox. However this high fruit dietary protocol will encourage healthy bowel movement and this should be sufficient, unless if you are at a chronic stage."

30. Today's Date:

Morning
(work towards continuing your night time dry fast up until at least 12pm)

Afternoon
(get hydrating with fresh fruit or even better slow juiced fruits/berries/melons)

Evening
(aim to wind down to a dry fast by around 6pm to 7pm)

Night
(work your way up to dry fasting from the evening until 12pm the following day)

Today's Notes (Highlights, Thoughts, Feelings, What Could You Improve On?)

"You can have your iris' read by an iridologist that works with Dr Bernard Jensen's system. An Iris Diagnosis will offer you information on specific areas of weakness that pre-exist for you to focus on."